Disclaimer

All the material contained in this book is provided for educational and informational purposes only. No responsibility can be taken for any results or outcomes resulting from the use of this material.

While every attempt has been made to provide information that is both accurate and effective, the author does not assume any responsibility for the misuse/misunderstood use of this information.

Author: Dr Mohammad Shariq Siddiqui (PT),

MPT (Master of Physical Therapy, Neurology)

MBA (Healthcare and Hospital Administration)

Fall Prevention Guide for Elderly

TABLE OF CONTENTS

Fall Prevention Guide for Elderly

Introduction

1 in 4 American aged 65+ falls each year. Every 11 seconds, an older adult is treated in the emergency room for a fall; every 19 minutes, an older adult die from a fall.

Falls are the leading cause of fatal injury and the most common cause of nonfatal trauma-related hospital admissions among older adults. Falls result in more than 2.8 million injuries treated in emergency departments annually, including over 800,000 hospitalizations and more than 27,000 deaths.

The statistic is from Centers for Disease Control and Prevention, USA. Unites States being a large, first world country is a good sample for the rest of world. In some ways this is representative of many societies with similar lifestyles.

Most falls will not result in a serious injury. However, half of the people who fall, will have repeated falls (NHS, UK), subsequently in the time to come. That leads to a fear of falling which may further lead the people to getting withdrawn. They tend to lose their confidence and avoid moving often. They need support for carrying out their daily chores that involve moving around.

So, the **falls significantly affect their independence.** Therefore, it is important to nip the problem in the bud. This will not only have a physical but a significant positive mental health impact.

Fall Prevention Guide for Elderly

Unfortunately, many older people accept their condition as a natural process of their ageing. They do not believe that it is possible to improve their health condition, their present situation and also get stronger so that they can be more stable.

Interestingly, **the reality is that falls can be prevented**. A recent study published in the American Journal of Preventive Medicine (Volume 55, issue 3, September 2018, pages 290-297) showed that just a single fall intervention like vitamin d supplementation, medication management or home modification could prevent falls and avert medical costs.

Therefore, it is all the more important to be careful with certain age groups with specific conditions to take care of themselves and prevent the falls. Small efforts suggested in this book to prevent a fall that can lead to a major mishap or can cause mental agony associated with reduced independence sometimes happening after a fall.

Chapter 1: What is ageing?

Does my age number determine my risk of fall?

Fall chances certainly increases with age. Does that mean a specific number of years lived will simply define your risk of falling?

Certainly, it is not that simple!

Let us first understand the concept of aging before understanding the depth of the reasons for fall. For doing that we need to understand how to define being old. Who is an older person? With the advent of newer healthcare technologies to diagnose, treat diseases, along with improved disease understanding. The lifespan of an average person is increasing. Many people are living up to 80 and 90 years, some may even live longer. Do everyone age similarly. The answer is obvious NO.

Many people remain fully functional and do a full-time job even in their 70s. You can see many of celebrities living that way.

Are they not ageing? Of course, they are. We cannot say by just looking at a number that someone is too old or too young. Many time doctors describe in their note that a person looks younger than his chronological age or vice versa. What does that mean? It means that apart from looking at age from a quantitative aspect, you need to look at it from a qualitative aspect as well.

Fall Prevention Guide for Elderly

This qualitative aspect can help look the process of ageing in a different way. Qualitative aspect means looking at your health status at a particular age is more important than just looking at your number of years lived. I am not demotivating people who are young and have diseases. My point is to convey a concept that the way you live your life may affect your body and ultimately the way it ages. This fundamental understanding can and should change the perspectives. Positivity might enter with the feeling to control the notion of uncontrolled process of ageing. People may focus more on their qualitative health which will be a welcome trend.

Science also backs up the fact that people who are more active in their lives experience slow rate of decline in their mobility. Being active will also help prevent chronic diseases like diabetes mellitus and hypertension. Let us have a look at one classification of aging which is based on the same premise.

Aging can be of 2 types:

1. **Primary Aging**: is the natural aspect of development. A person will have some reduction in the abilities with time like reduction in bone mass, some degree of hearing or vision loss. It is a slow process.

2. **Secondary Aging** is the aging due to diseases process and poor health practices. These includes no exercise, smoking, excess body weight due to

Fall Prevention Guide for Elderly

high caloric intake etc. This is often preventable, whether through lifestyle choice or modern medicine.

People with better health practices like exercise, non-sedentary lifestyle, healthy diet and less stressful life can slow secondary aging effectively. This may also have some positive effect on the primary aging process. To what degree that is determined by your genes may remain complex?

However, there is no doubt that if a person ages both ways primary as well as secondary then he or she will have a worse health given a particular age. Your life may be a steep fall from a cliff if you are aging both ways. On the other hand, primary aging with a better health and lifestyle may help you remain independent up to a greater number of our chronological age.

Therefore, it must be an important focus area which we need to keep in mind. In addition, it is also a reminder to not look at age just as a numeral, it is true that age is just a number. People like Edwina Brocklesby or Eddy Diget or Gwyn Haslock have been athletes in their 70s.

What matters more is the quality of aging which you need to keep up with and is quite possible to achieve. This will help change our mind set to effectively gain some level of control that is otherwise inevitably taken away from the aging process.

Fall Prevention Guide for Elderly

Chapter 2 -What is Balance/Imbalance?

How any physical body does balance itself?

A Human body is like any other physical body. All the principles of gravity acting on any physical body are also applicable on the human body. Any physical body on which gravity is acting will have 3 things:

1. **Center of Gravity**: It also has its center of gravity which is an imaginary point on a physical body where gravity acts on it. For a human body, that point exists near the lower back.

2. **Line of Gravity**: The line of gravity is an imaginary vertical line from the center of gravity to the ground.

3. **Base of Support:** Base of support refers to the area under an object. The area includes every point of contact that the object makes with the supporting surface. In easy language it means the area under your body.

For any person or physical body to remain stable, his/her line of gravity should remain within his/her base of support.

Therefore, balance is the ability of a human body to maintain its line of gravity over its base of support.

Similarly, imbalance is the inability to maintain the line of gravity of human body over its base of support. Leaning tower of pizza is still balancing itself because its line of gravity is within its base of support.

So is the case with a human body, it will be stable until its line of gravity will remain within its base of support.

A human body is certainly a physical body however it is also a live entity with its different segments moving and changing its shape in different positions from standing to stooping to lying on the bed. This makes the human body quite different also from any physical body which is having a constant shape and size.

Furthermore, a human being is a bipedal living entity which means contrary to its quadruped or 4-legged fellow living relatives. Its base of support is much narrower.

If you allow me to compare it with a non-living being, I will say a human being is like a moving tower with only 2 legs. It is more challenging to balance a physical moving tower which is changing its shape many times in a day, yet it does not fall.

What an incredible physical body!

However, there is lot more happening in the background for a human body to balance itself. Let us find out how that happens in a simple way next!

How Does Human Body perform the function of Balance?

Balance is achieved by our body in a fascinating way. As explained earlier the human body is a moving and shape changing physical body. In addition, it walks and moves on a narrow base i.e. on its 2 legs. Therefore, it needs constant update about its positioning and constant response based on its position to control itself. Several body systems work constantly to do this function.

The major sense organs that do the function of providing awareness of different body segments to the brain:

1. Inner Ear
2. Joint and muscle nerves
3. Eyes

Brain receives all the inputs constantly for body positioning from the above sense organs. It interprets it by complex processes within itself. Then provide responses in the form of signals to our muscles to control and balance the body on its base of support.

Therefore, **muscles** are the end points where brain signal comes and muscle work accordingly sometimes by relaxation and sometimes by contraction to keep the body balanced. See the diagram below.

Fall Prevention Guide for Elderly

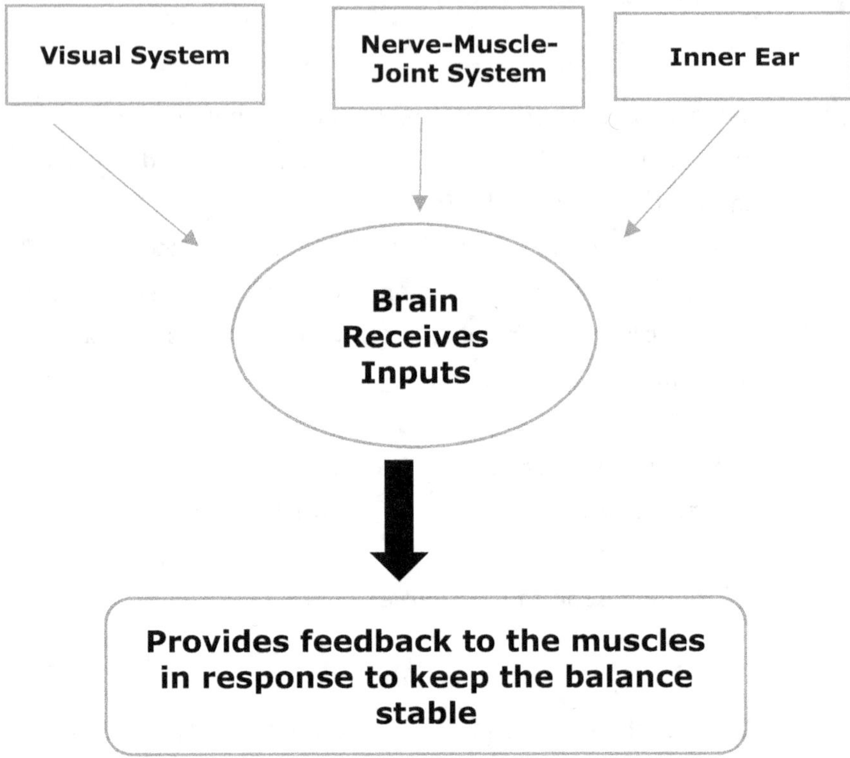

This is a simplified form of balance mechanism, but it sheds light on the body systems which work together to keep us balanced.

This mechanism is active all the time and in all the positions. Whether you are standing, running, dancing or even sleeping.

This system is constantly protecting you from imbalance. Of course, the visual system may not be helping you while sleeping but that is ok because you ensure that you are well balanced when you sleep. The constant interplay of these body system is the mechanism which ensures that you are remain stable when you change positions, when you walk or run or when you trip or stumble.

Therefore, the functional and physical integrity of these body systems including inner ear, eyes and joint muscle complex is key to have a good balance.

Chapter 3: Why do some older people fall?

Human body ensures that you are well balanced in the most difficult positions as well. However sometimes we can fall, and some people tend to fall more. Let us understand why?

There are several factors which causes people to fall. These includes:

Environmental Factors:

- **Slippery Floor**: Commonly falls occur in places where there is little friction like bathrooms, passages with reduced frictions or slick floors. It's a common occurrence that many people fall in bathrooms or wet floors.

- **Unfamiliar surroundings:** A person who old and weak may be fine in his home yet one fine day after changing home settings he or she might fall. This is because of the confusion and extra mental burden on the mind of someone who is already having weak senses or muscle system to maintain the balance.

- **Dim light:** Most common mistake due to which people often fall is the dim light. Vision along with other joint sensations act as cue for body to maintain balance. If lighting is not adequate it may challenge someone who is prone to fall. This ultimately can cause a fall and injury associated with it. Therefore, adequate lighting is very fundamental step to control the fall.

Weakness and Frailty:

Weakness we all must have heard is a feeling of low energy. This is a subjective feeling of low energy, yet it may have several physical reasons for it like low hemoglobin, low blood protein levels or vitamin deficiencies. All such causes need to be first identified and appropriately treated by the medical professionals.

Next comes frailty which is a broader clinical concept defined as the decline in functions of various body systems. It is defined by features like slow walking speed, low physical activity, low energy, weak grip strength and unexplained weight loss. All of which predisposes a person to fall when faced with fall prone circumstances.

Visual and Hearing Impairments

As discussed in the last chapter, balance is achieved by body via interpreting various sensations from the body senses including vision, muscle-joints systems, and inner ear. Then after making sense of these sensations, body activates muscles to achieve balance. This process takes place within seconds. Therefore, our senses like vision, joint sensations are important aspect of achieving a good balance.

When there is a visual impairment. This impairment may be in the form of cataract in people after a certain age or any other visual disease. This reduces the capacity of our body to know the relative position of its different parts in space by means of vision. Now a human being who is already old, weak is having reduced vision is like a weak soldier with one lesser arsenal of arms. This makes someone even more prone to fall.

Inner ear as we all know is important for balance and any disease which affect them can affect balance. That is why even a young person with inner ear disease experience dizziness and vertigo. Inner ear diseases like BPPV or Meniere's disease therefore affect balance.

Although hearing may not be having a direct role in balance and stability. Interestingly, **even hearing loss may make someone more prone to falls**. There are many explanations for it.

One of the explanations is that when someone is not hearing, he or she is not aware of his surroundings. Therefore, someone with poor hearing may get surprised and misbalanced due to that.

Other plausible explanation is the **cognitive overload**. This means because when someone is not hearing normally, his brain is working extra hard to compensate the hearing loss. This reduces the brain capacity for other work like being aware of body position and providing directions to the muscles for balance which might cause imbalance and fall.

Low Levels of Vitamin D:

Low levels of vitamin D is a risk for both falls and fractures, and supplementing with vitamin D by the medical care giver is shown to significantly reduce the risk of both.

Vitamin D is important for muscle function and the deficiency of Vitamin D can cause muscle weakness. Muscles are the key component in body movement, coordination, and balance.

Their weakness is a risk for balance impairment. Therefore, if anyone feels risk of falls, he or she must have Vitamin D levels checked. If deficient or insufficient the under medical supervision, they must be supplemented with the best possible route of administration. Lastly there are enough evidence to prove that vitamin d deficiency can increase the risk of fall while treating the deficiency leads to a reduction in it.

Nerve Muscle and Joint Impairments

Muscles, joints, and nerves function together in a human body also known as neuromuscular system.

Fall Prevention Guide for Elderly

This system is most critical system working to balance the human body. Beginning from their role in picking up sensations of different body parts via nerves inside joint and muscles. This system of nerve muscle and joints also is a response system. This means your brain provide the muscles a signal via specific nerves to balance the body on its base of support depending on the position of the body. This is the reason why brain stroke affect muscles and movements.

Reflexes are the basic reaction to sudden inputs like if I hit your knee joint with a medical hammer. Your knee will instantaneously bend without even your conscious effort. This is a muscle or joint reflex. These reflexes also serve you for balance. You may realize while travelling in a car or train that when you are asleep, and you unconsciously stoop too much or bend your neck too much. Your muscles instantaneously correct the excess bending or stooping sometimes with a bit of gentle jerk. This is a muscle reflex mechanism which protects yourself even when you are sleeping in a moving car.

Muscles reflexes slows with age. This is more so in people who don't train their muscles or do exercises for muscle maintenance.

In addition, diseases like arthritis, ankle sprain, muscle strain or any other complication of different diseases (like diabetes neuropathy) affecting the nerve muscle joint system may predispose you to fall.

Medications side effects

Many older people commonly take medications for sleep disorders, anxiety, depression, high BP or chronic pain or any other specific disease.

Some of these medicines may have side effects which can affect the ability of the body to maintain a steady balance.

Therefore, it is best for the doctors as well as patients to keep in mind the risk of falls when prescribing such medications. An easy way is to screen the patient for risk of fall. In case a doctor forgets that, the patient must remind and confirm if the medication is safe and will not increase the chances of fall.

In case patient realizes it later that the medicines are making him or her unsteady. He or she should immediately inform the prescribing physician.

Sometimes the effect wanes off after certain initial doses. However, if that effect stays, it is best recommended for the physician to either change medication or reduce doses of medication else completely stop the medicine causing unsteadiness. The principle in medical prescription is that the benefit of any medicine must outweigh the risk.

Dizziness/Orthostatic/Postural Hypotension

Orthostatic hypotension is defined as the drop in blood pressure upon standing. Therefore, it is also known as postural hypotension.

Symptoms: Orthostatic hypotension may cause dizziness, light headedness, weakness, or fainting, which can either lead to instability or a fall altogether.

The drop in blood pressure in orthostatic hypotension **may be sudden** or **within 3 minutes of standing up** which is a case in classical orthostatic hypotension.

It is defined as a fall in systolic blood pressure (the upper reading of blood pressure) of at least 20 mm Hg or diastolic blood pressure (lower reading of blood pressure) of at least 10 mm Hg when a person assumes a standing position.

The REASON why it occurs is that the normal constriction (normal narrowing) of the lower body blood vessels, is either delayed or absent.

As a result, **blood pools in the blood vessels of the legs for a longer period and less amount of blood is returned to the heart**. This reduces the blood reaching the heart and in turn lesser blood is supplied to the brain. This cause fainting, dizziness, or lightheadedness. Sometimes it can even happen to some normal persons if he or she suddenly stands up after prolonged sitting or rest.

In the later part of the book, we will also find out the possible solutions to the problem.

Foot related Factors

Human feet are the body part bearing immense pressure especially when someone is in weight bearing position or moving around. Many feet ailments like bunion (the great toe deformity) or foot muscle weakness or heel spurs are common in old age. They impact the foot mechanics meaning that they may affect how force is taken up by feet and distributed. This faulty distribution may affect balance leading to falls.

History of Falls

An elderly person who has experienced few falls in the past may develop fear of falling, which leads to reduced confidence. This may also lead to confinement, impaired confidence in the capacity to do normal daily activities, isolation, depressive moods, and reduced quality of life.

With these factors along with fear of falling, the person may function at lower than actual capacity which further reduces the abilities of the person making him/her become prone to falling.

Diseases affecting Balance

There are diseases which directly can affect balance of a person. Common ones include knee or hip Osteoarthritis, Rheumatoid Arthritis, Parkinson's disease, Peripheral neuropathies etc. Taking common example of arthritis, people suffering from it have stiff joints, weak muscles or other associated impairments leading to difficulty in walking and stabilizing themselves in walking. Similarly, in Parkinson's disease, a person may become rigid, have tremors and is slow in movement and reactions. When such a person walks, there are chances that there may be instability or inability to properly balance if there is any external challenge like something is scattered on the floor.

Neuropathies are nerve diseases which can affect the nerves providing signal about body positioning or the nerves bringing signal from the brain to the muscles for control.

In all these diseases, treating them is foremost thing which needs to be done. In addition, exercises described in chapter 6 can additionally help.

Chapter 4: How likely you are to fall?

Let's find out if you are at high risk

Finding out the risk to falling for any person is an essential step towards fall prevention. Looking at the statistics of falls indicates higher incidences of falls in the elderly especially post 65 years or with chronic diseases affecting balance. It is imperative to conduct a fall assessment and find out if someone is at high risk for falling. This will prevent so much of mental, financial loss as well as suffering for anyone.

Let's begin!

All older people can be screened for fall risk. Each person needs to be asked these 3 questions:

1. **Have you fallen in the past year?**
   a. If yes, how many times did you fall? and
   b. Were you inured when you fell?
2. **Do you feel unsteady when standing or walking?**
   a. Yes/No
3. **Do you worry about falling?**
   a. Yes/No

<u>If the answer is NO to all the 3 questions then the person is at low risk for falling.</u>

On the other hand, if the answer is yes to any of the 3 questions then further the timed up and go test needs to be done. You can take help from one of your family member/friends who is healthy and confident to support you in case of instability or imbalance. In addition, who can also keep a tab on time.

Timed Up and Go Test

Materials needed for this test:
1.   One Chair with Arm Rest
2.   Stopwatch
3.   Marker to mark 3 meters

How to do this Timed Up and Go Test
- **You need to sit on the chair having arm rest**
- **Ask your family member or friend to draw a line or put a mark 3 meters distance away from the chair**
- **Ask him to start the stop, then stand up and walk naturally up to the 3 meters mark**
- **Turn around just past the 3-meter mark and come back and sit on the chair**
- **Try not to take the help of your hands while getting up or sitting**
- **Make sure your chair is stable enough**
- **Make sure the person keeping the stopwatch stops the time when you sit back**
- **You can use assistive device if you are using it in the day to day walking.**
- **You can also see the video of it on YouTube for demo. Just search Timed up and go test.**

If you took 14 seconds or long, then you are at high risk for falling otherwise a low risk.

Above assessment is taken up from by CDC's (USA) STEADI (Stopping Elderly Accidents, Deaths, and Injuries Initiative) although that involves some additional steps.

Functional Reach and Multidirectional Reach Tests

These tests check the person's ability to reach in different directions as far as possible without stepping out. These are generally done by a physical therapists or other medical experts. You can discuss it with your family physician if you want to check your multidirectional stability. In chapter 6 we have given certain exercises to improve multidirectional stability. These will improve your multidirectional abilities regardless of the testing.

Last but not the least, you must also get your hearing and vision assessment done to ensure that it is not making you prone to fall.

Chapter 5: Way to Recovery-Interventions for Fall Reduction

Most important for anyone with high risk for falling is to understand that no matter how weak you think you are or how inactive you have been, **you can ALWAYS improve your situation.**

Never underestimate the power of small positive daily action that accumulate over time. Consistent and conscientious action is a force to be reckoned with.

Let's begin!

- Make your home environment safer.

  1. Remove things you can increases your chance to stumble like shoes, clothes etc. from the places you walk.

  2. Remove any stuff which increases your chance of tripping like small throw rugs

  3. Keep items in places in approach. Sometimes people use stool to reach certain items making themselves vulnerable.

  4. Have some support handles in the bathroom safely and strategically placed to provide the support.

  5. Improve the lighting in your home. Often dim light will prevent you from seeing clearly and may increase the risk of tripping and falling.

  6. Wear well fitted shoes with appropriate cushioning. Often people order shoes online and they compromise on fitting. This may put them

on risk of falling. Footwear with good grip and fitting may help you walk with great stability.

- Orthostatic hypotension

    1. As discussed, **orthostatic hypotension is defined as the drop in blood pressure upon standing. Therefore, it is also known as postural hypotension. This might cause someone to fall**.

    2. The drop in blood pressure **may be sudden** or **within 3 minutes of standing up** which is classical orthostatic hypotension.

    3. It occurs predominantly by delayed (or absent) constriction (normal narrowing) of the lower body blood vessels, which is normally required to maintain an adequate blood pressure when changing position to standing. Less blood goes into the organs and muscles which makes someone to fall more likely. You can request your primary care physician to evaluate your BP from sit to stand. Otherwise, you may also check yourself at home by measuring your blood pressure from sit to stand **and** find out if you have orthostatic hypotension.

Common symptoms of Orthostatic Hypotension

Many people may have no symptoms of it while others have different symptoms which may include

    1. Headache/ Blurriness in vision

2. Lightheadedness
3. Feeling of about to fall/pass out
4. Weakness or fatigue
5. Nausea or hot

When do these symptoms more likely to happen

1. In the morning especially when you get up

2. After a large meal

3. When you get anxious

4. When you are straining on the toilet

5. When you are ill

Orthostatic hypotension can be caused by or may be linked with

1. Diabetes
2. Certain BP medications
3. High BP
4. Dehydration
5. Diseases like Parkinson's disease and Dementia

What can you do to reduce orthostatic hypotension?

1. Inform your healthcare provider if you think you are having orthostatic hypotension who first needs to review the medications you are taking

2. Be slow when you get up from your bed, especially in the morning. Since this blood pressure lowering happens because of pooling of blood in the legs. Give your body some time to adjust by keep sitting on the bed for some time before standing up (few minutes).

3. Before getting up, do some simple exercises like remaining on the edge of the bed, move your hands up down. Also, while remain sitting on the bed, move your knee back and forth.

4. Do some of the activities like bathing sitting on a chair. Bathroom falls are a usual occurrence and orthostatic hypotension may be one of the factors.

5. Make sure you have some support around when you stand up.

6. Avoid taking very hot water showers. This increase the skin blood flow and might reduce the blood pressure causing someone to experience orthostatic hypotension more likely.

7. Stay Hydrated, drink enough of fluids during the day unless you have a medical condition that restricts fluid intake.

8. Try sleeping with a pillow that raises head level. You may also use a wedge pillow or raise bed end after consulting and taking consent from your physician.

9. Do not walk unless you feel stable

- **Vitamin D Deficiency & Treatment**

Several researches indicate that low levels of vitamin D are associated with increased risks of falls and reduction in muscle strength and muscle mass in the elderly population.

Fall Prevention Guide for Elderly

Therefore, if consuming daily recommended dosage of Vitamin D, will help in reducing the future risk of falls.

Vitamin D is made by our skin when UVB-irradiation from summer sunshine falls on it. Vitamin D to a small extent is also received by absorption from food. **However, these processes become less efficient with age**. Therefore, sunshine exposure may not be making adequate levels of Vitamin D for you especially in older age.

Loss of mobility or non-availability of sun exposure especially in low-income countries may further increase the chances of deficiency. Reduced appetite and financial problems often add to these problems.

Thus, low levels of Vitamin D are common world-wide, but is more common and more severe in older people.

Daily doses of 600 IU/day for adults and 800 IU/day for those at risk or over 70 years old is recommended. However, it is recommended to check your Vitamin D levels and ensure that you are not deficient for Vitamin D. In addition, before administering vitamin d make sure that it is a nonprescription medicine at this dose in your country. In several countries the Vitamin D pills up to 5000 IU are non-prescription or over the counter medicine. Therefore, you can start with such a dose without prescription if you have normal levels of Vitamin D and thus maintain your levels of it. Some countries like Finland introduced food fortification and they have virtually abolished deficiency in most parts of the population.

Fall Prevention Guide for Elderly

If you are found deficient for Vitamin D, then a greater dosage will be required and may need a prescription from your doctor.

Annual Vision and Hearing examination

Eyes provide very crucial inputs about the body position in space to the brain. However, the diseases or any visual impairment affecting the normal vision may also affect the balance and coordination of the body. This might lead to an increased risk of falling.

Therefore, get an eye examination done once in a year to find out if the glasses need to be updated or not. Also, if there are any diseases like Cataract which is common after a certain age.

Attempt by the eye doctor to find out the initial signs of eye diseases. Common example is the increased intraocular pressure which might be a risk factor for glaucoma.

Annual hearing examination as part of normal annual health check

As discussed in the chapter 3 that one reason for fall could be hearing loss. Therefore, it is important to identify and correct the hearing loss by the appropriate treatment. At best, a visit to an ENT doctor can be made. Otherwise, a general physician may also do a basic hearing screen to find out if you have hearing loss and need further treatment by a consulting ear specialist or audiologist.

Chapter 6: Work on Muscle system: Home Exercise to Improve Strength and Balance

According to research, exercises that increases the strength in the muscles improves balance in the older adults. Strength training of the **leg**, **back** as well as **core muscles** improves the fall risk as well as quality of life. The weakness of muscles of the leg is an independent risk factor for fall.

The exercise mentioned here are very simple and are low-moderate intensity meaning that they should not cause too much demand on your body. You can also start with few exercises initially and progress as you feel more confident. However, if you are in doubt or feel unwell to start this exercise program, you can always consult your doctor to find out if you can participate in the prescribed exercise program.

Warm up:

Warm up before any exercise program is necessary since the muscles at rest may not have enough blood supply. Warm up will increase the blood supply and prepare muscles for effective exercises.

You warm up should be at least 3-5 minutes of light exercises.

These light exercises may include:

- Stationary cycle

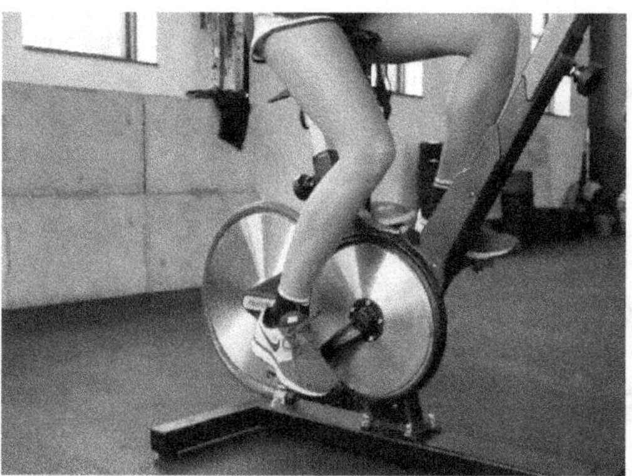

- Arm Movements up down in the front.

- Trunk Swings while sitting

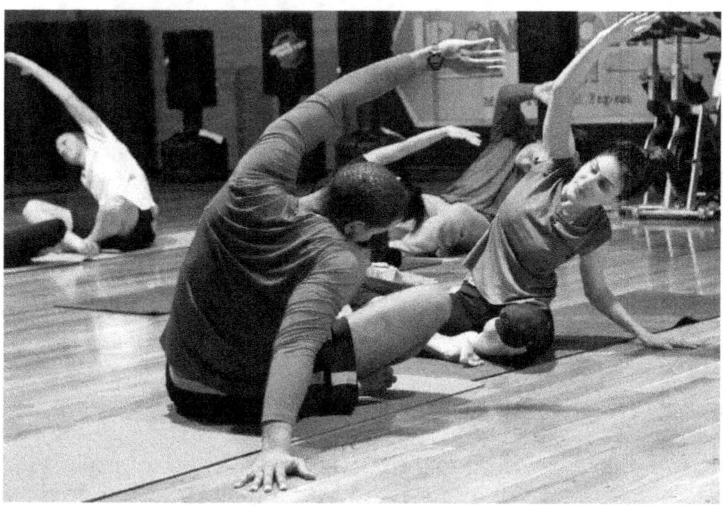

- Shoulder Shrugs (shoulder movement up/down) while sitting

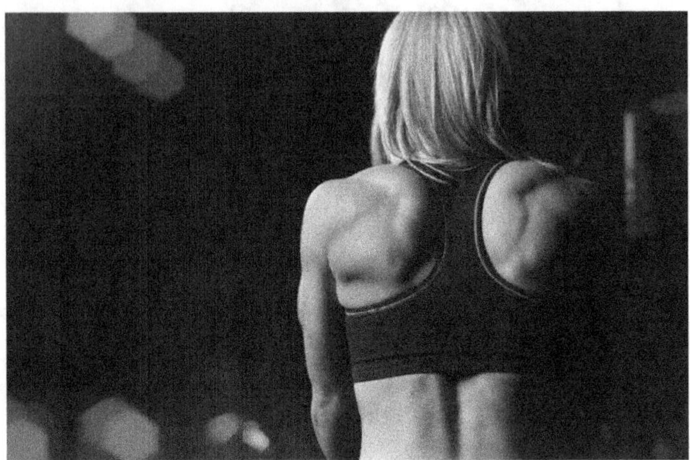

- Alternate Knee lifts during sittings
- Wrist Circles
- Ankle Circles

Walking

Walking for at least 20-30 minutes per day at your usual pace. You may break it down to smaller intervals like 10 minutes' walk three times a day. It is preferable to do these before meals or 2 hours after meals. If you are doing it before meals, make sure that you are well hydrated and not low on energy or sugar.

Stretching: Often Ignored Intervention

Let me share my personal experience with one of my patients who had dementia and had a history of fall with minor skin bruises. This patient was not aware of his actions and surroundings due to advanced dementia. He could not even speak and understand any command due to advanced dementia.

It was difficult to make him exercise.

However, after examination I found that his calf muscles

were tight and may be pushing him backward to make him unsteady. Calf muscles are located at the back of your lower legs. When I manually stretched his calves, his fall rate reduced drastically. This made me realize the importance of flexibility in reducing falls.

Therefore, you must self-stretch or get someone gently stretch your calves and hamstrings. Let us see how:

Calf (leg) stretch- (see diagram)

1. Stand against a wall keeping an arm's length of distance with the wall.
2. Take support of the wall in front by placing your hands on the wall.
3. Now place one foot ahead and other behind but both need to be in line.

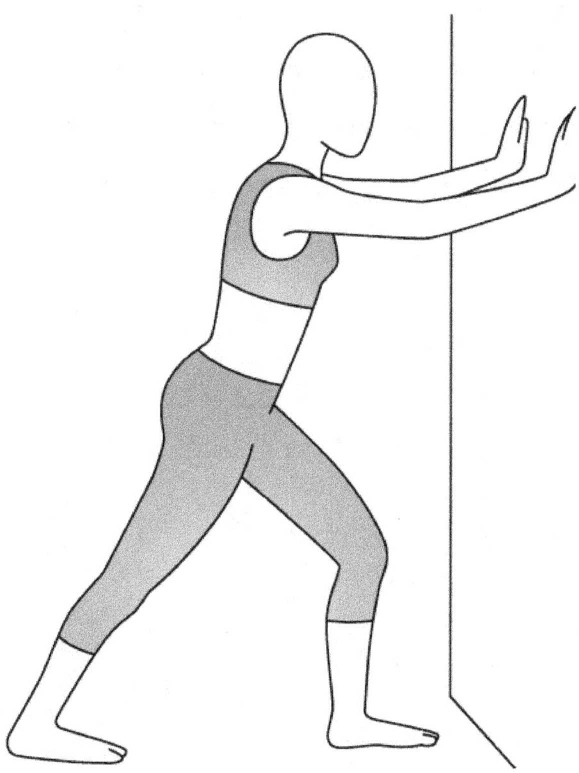

4. The rear knees should be straight while gradually bending the front knee.
5. Bend your front knee gradually while keeping your back straight while taking your hip region towards the wall.
6. Stop bending your front knee at the point where you can no more bend it while the stretch at the back of your feet is quite sufficient for you to bear.
7. The heel of the rear foot should remain in contact with the ground.
8. Stay in that stretched position for some time (10-15 seconds).
9. Later bring the other foot backwards and repeat the stretch on the other leg.

Hamstring (Thigh) Stretch (See Diagram)

1. Sit on your bed comfortably with both knees straight. You can have a back support of a wall or head end of your bed.
2. Now try to touch your toes without bending your knees.
3. This should have a stretch feel at the back of your thighs.
4. Stay in that stretched position for some time (10-15 seconds).

5. Repeat it few more times. Slowly increase the time of you feel the stretch but ensure that you do not bear excessive pain. Only a bit of stretch pain is fine.

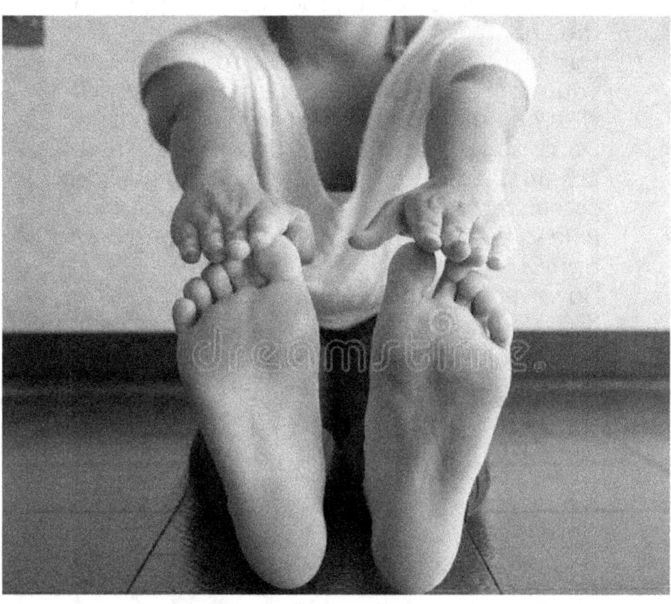

Alternately:

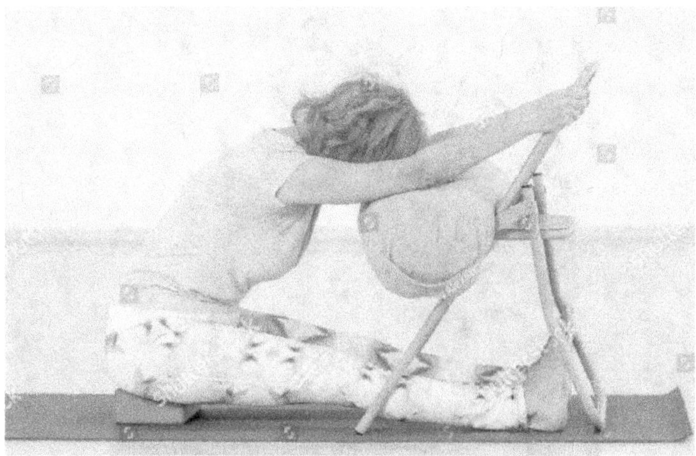

Trunk Stretches for Improved Mobility:

1. Sitting comfortably on a chair with knees hanging down.
2. Rotate yourself trying to grab the upper end of the chair.
3. Initially you may not be able to do, however as you progress it will become more approachable with one day you may touch and grab it.
4. Do not overdo or touch it on the first day if you are unable or are overweight. Keep yourself comfortable.
5. Pain is a guide if it is very painful then do not try it.
6. However, if you can do it comfortably, it will help you in many ways including improving your lung health by making your trunk more flexible to expand.

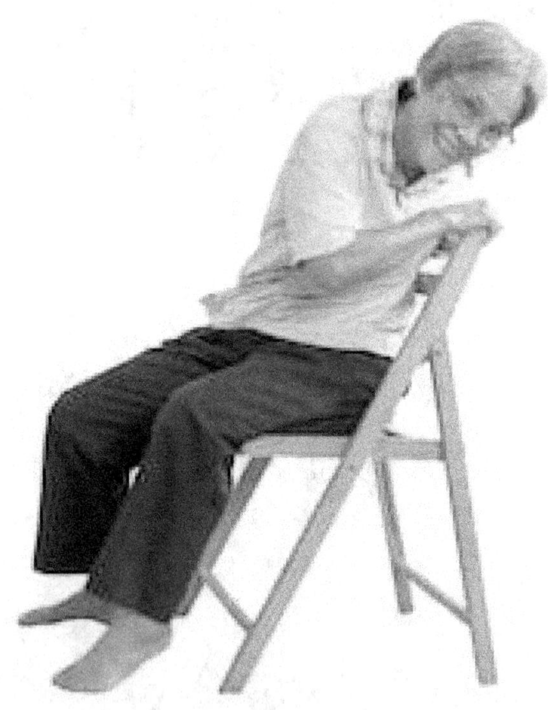

Strength Exercises for Balance

1. **Straight Leg raises**
   a. Start with a lying on your back facing the ceiling.
   b. Raise one leg slightly up to 6 inches from the bed surface.
   c. Hold it for 3-5 second at the end.
   d. Be slow in this exercise.
   e. Now the exercise with the other leg.
   f. Do 2 sets on each leg with each set having 7-10 repetitions.
   g. It is more important to do exercises correctly then to repeat it for a higher number of times.
   h. You can take break in between the sets. A good way to check if your exercise intensity is within limits is to ensure that you can talk comfortably while exercising. If you can talk while exercises, then you are doing a moderate intensity exercise which means your heart lung system is working within moderate level and not exerting excessively.

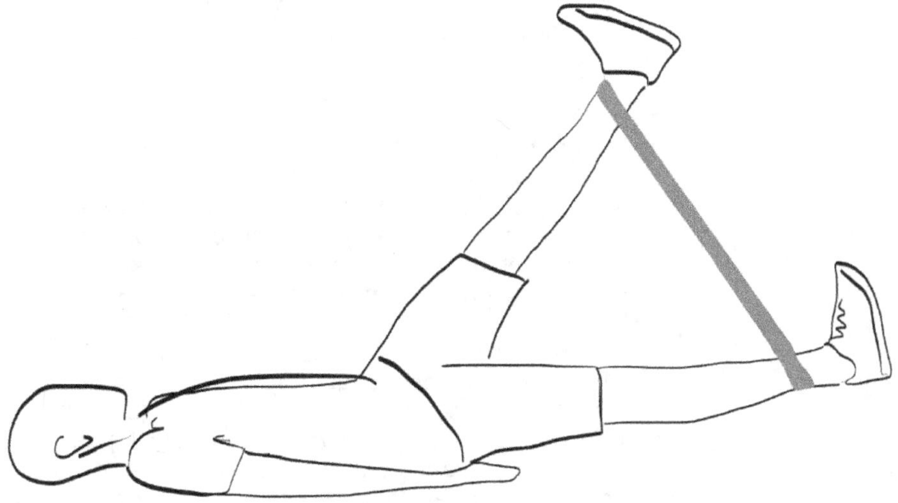

2. **Side Leg Raises (Similar to the above exercise)**
    a. Start with a side lying position on your bed.
    b. Bend the knee of the leg which is touching the bed surface
    c. Bring the upper leg just behind the lower leg.
    d. Start lifting the upper leg from here up to 30 degrees or as much as you can.
    e. Be slow in this exercise.
    f. Never hold your breath, keeping breathing normally.
    g. Bring the leg back to its initial position.
    h. Make sure your toes are in the horizontal plane.
    i. Now turn to the other side and repeat the exercise with the other leg.
    j. Do 2 sets on each leg with each set having 7-10 repetitions.
    k. It is more important to do exercises correctly then to repeat it for a higher number of times.
    l. You can take break in between the sets. A good way to check if your exercise intensity is within limits is to ensure that you can talk comfortably while exercising. If you can talk while exercises, then you are doing a moderate intensity exercise which means your heart lung system is working within moderate level and not exerting excessively.

3. **Mini Squats**
    a. Keep your feet 12-18 inches apart.
    b. Bend your knees little bit.
    c. Keep you back either straight or if you can comfortably do then just bend a bit forward to recruit the back of the hip muscle known as gluteus maximum which is often weak as we age.
    d. Do the squats in this position as a set of 7-10 repetitions or just as much as you can do. Do 2 sets in total.
    e. Do not go very deep by bending your knees into excessive angles. Bend in such a way so that your knees do not cross your great toes.
    f. You can also watch the same on YouTube for demo.

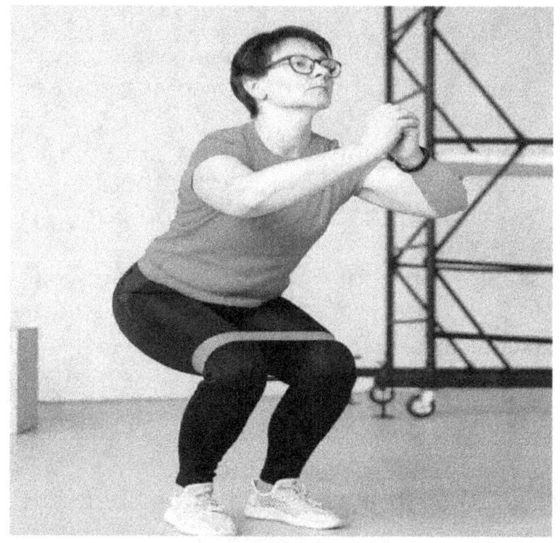

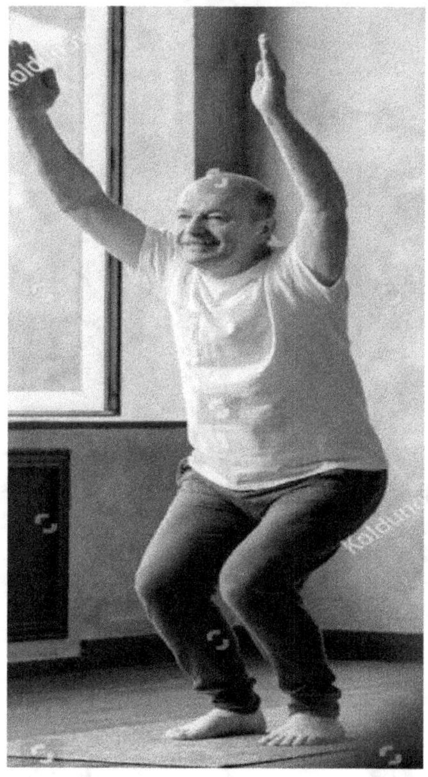

4. **Sitting knee straitening exercise with/without weight cuff.**
    a. Sit comfortably on the bed/chair while both your legs hanging by the bed/chair and feet above the ground.
    b. You can tie a weight cuff of 1 kg to begin with initially else you can start without weight and later add weight as you get more comfortable.
    c. Now straighten your knees completely while keeping your back straight and not leaning backwards.
    d. Repeat it 10-15 times in each set. Do a total of 2 sets.
    e. Take a break in between and make sure you can talk comfortably while doing this exercise to ensure moderate intensity level.

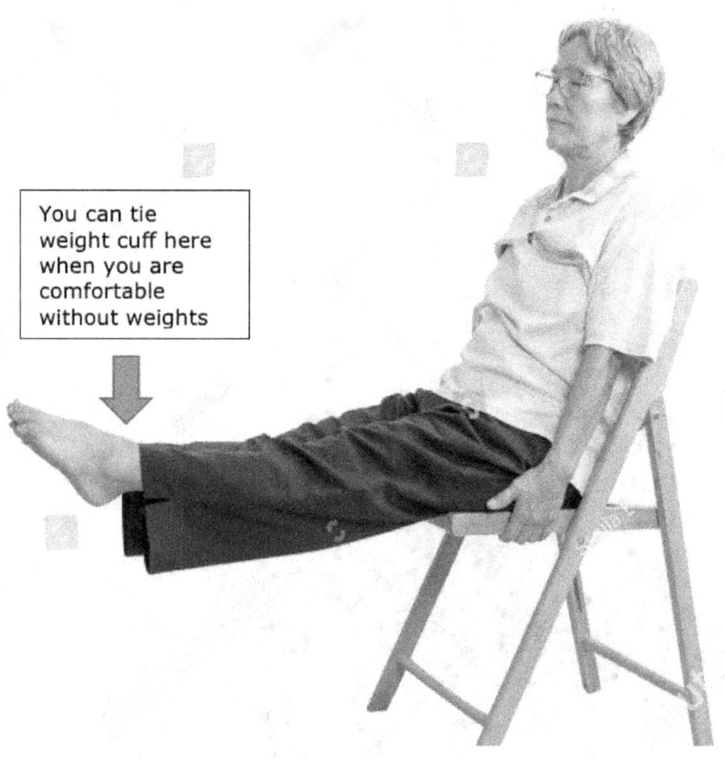

Some other additional modified sitting exercises you can do:

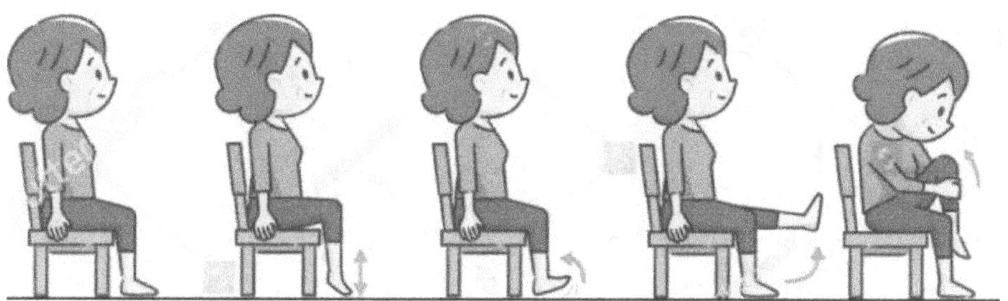

5. **Sit to Stand with 2 hands**
    a.   With 2 hands support stand up from a chair and then sit down
    b.   Make sure the chair is stable or will not move while you stand or sit.

6. **Sit to Stand with one hand and no hands support**
    a.   Start it when you feel you can do it comfortably with 2 hands
    b.   Do it with one hand support first
    c.   If you cannot control with one hand then do not try it now.

Static Balance Training

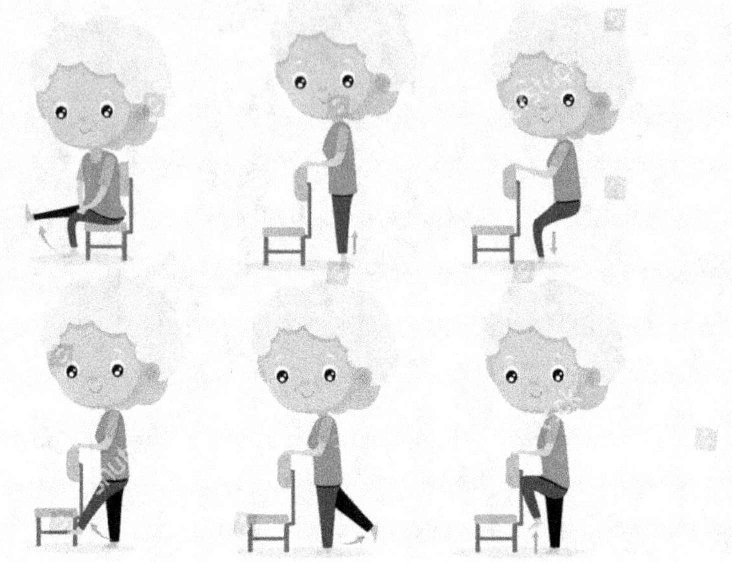

Fall Prevention Guide for Elderly

Step ups are one of the most important balance exercises that you can do to improve your mobility. Step up involve just rising one step at a staircase and then coming back to the original position. You can hold the handrail initially but as your balance improves, you can step up without holding any handrails.

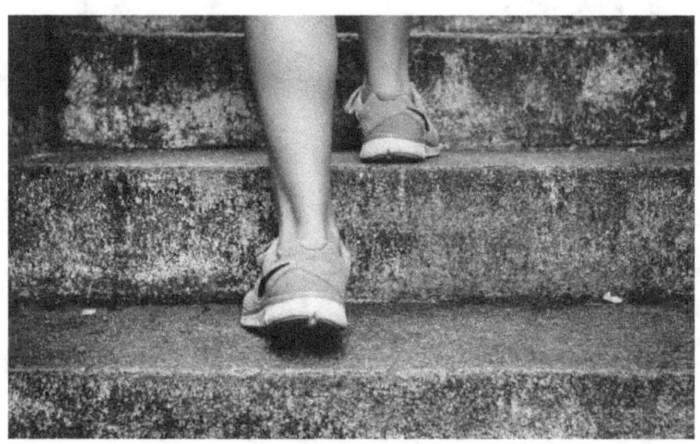

Dynamic Balance Training

Dynamic balance training as the name suggest is the balance training when your body is moving around. Once you are comfortable with static balance training. Add dynamic balance training in your schedule.

Side walking

A. Stand with your feet slightly apart.
B. Then start moving sideways in a slow and controlled manner.
C. When you complete 10-15 steps, return.
D. You can do it alongside a wall initially if you do not feel confident enough. You can walk sideways facing the wall.
E. Once you feel confident then do it with eyes closed. Make sure you have something close for support may be a family member.

Fall Prevention Guide for Elderly

Fall Prevention Guide for Elderly

Heel to Toe Walking

A. Place your left heel in front of your right big toe.
B. Then subsequently place your right heel in front of your left big toe.
C. This is a toe to toe walking.
D. You can also do it alongside a wall initially if you do not feel confident enough in the beginning.
E. Complete 10-15 steps, return in the reverse order.

Sideways Reach Tasks

1. Stand between a high and low table/platform positioned on either side.
2. Pick up objects from one table and transfer it to the other one
3. As you become more comfortable, increase the distance between the tables and increase the weight to be transferred between the tables. You may also increase or decrease the height of these tables.
4. These exercises will improve the multidirectional stability.

Ball Games

1. This will involve a family member, neighbor or a friend.
2. Use Inflated large balls which will be light.
3. Start catching/throwing them while sitting or standing with support from a wall or a person.
4. Catch/Throw the ball in different directions to improve multidirectional stability.
5. Add a mental task like naming a movie which has a specific famous film star or any general knowledge game.
6. This mental task will further increase the complexity of training.
7. After some time use smaller or harder balls.

Lost and Found Games

1. Request someone in the family or friend to play this game.
2. Ask the person, to hide certain object somewhere like under the bed or sofa
3. The place needs to be such that searching for it may involve bending, reaching activities.
4. You can modify it according to your current level of abilities and confidence.

Fall Prevention Guide for Elderly

The exercises above make a foundational home exercise program. One can start slowly with fewer exercises in the beginning and add exercises as days go by and learns previous exercises.

Reliable research like Cochrane review, have found that most effective balance trainings were those which were done 3 times a week for a duration of 3 months.

Therefore, my recommendation is also to reach a level when you do these exercises 3 times a week.

Chapter 7: Mobility Aids

Mobility aids or walking aids are one of several devices a person may be issued to improve their walking pattern, balance or safety and move independently.

Mobility aids increase the base of support for an individual making them more stable.

It is possible that many of you may already be using a walking aid like cane for many reasons including balance issues or arthritis or any other disease.

These mobility aids can also be a means of transferring weight from the upper limb i.e. your arm, forearm, and hand to the ground, reducing load on the lower extremity which are your thighs, legs and feet. This way some stress is reduced on the lower limbs i.e. your thighs, legs, and feet.

In this chapter we will look at the 3 types of mobility aids commonly used for balance and mobility improvement.

This is a sensitive topic many times and people refuse to use these canes and walkers. They feel that it makes them look
handicapped or dependent.

They feel that it is an insult and a sign of helplessness to use a cane or walker. They continue to suffer with reduced mobility or difficult mobility yet do not use them.

The reality is that a cane or a walker is not a sign of weakness. One should think in this way. These devices like cane are designed to help you. Using one effectively and helping yourself is a sign of being strong and independent.

If you need one, get it… and use it. Never ever regret growing old. It is a privilege denied to many.

Although one must always try to correct the causes of immobility first. For example, if your balance issues are due to factors described in the previous chapters and fall in the correctable categories. You should try to follow the interventions described above or possibly take specialist help like a trained physical therapist.

However, due to many other reasons affecting your mobility may not be completely correctable like chronic diseases. Therefore, your doctor/therapist decides to prescribe you one of these aids in your best interest. You must not think about these as sign of weakness rather an opportunity to regain your comfort and mobility.

Walking aids may fall into multiple categories like

1. **Walking Canes/Sticks**
Many of us may already know what these are. They are usually made of aluminum with one end being a handle and the other having a rubber tip. Many of these canes are adjustable (about 33 to 37 inches) and some may be foldable for convenience. When choosing a cane, make sure it is sturdy, yet lightweight and easy to carry.

The distal tip of canes should have rubber to prevent the walking aid from slipping. Some rubbers also have vacuum mechanism to have a firm grip on the ground. Therefore, the rubber should not be worn or cracked and should fit well onto the point of the walking aid.

2. **Walkers**
These provide more support and balance than canes. However, there is a greater social stigma to use these because they can provide greater support. Therefore, many older people prefer walking canes. In addition, cane are considered to have better social appeal and acceptance than walkers.

For people who need greater support may still require and prescribed a walker and there is no shame in it. It is the independence with the aid that can liberate you from dependence and improve your quality of life. People are never happy with us and thus you must not care of what people will say.

3. **Elbow Crutches/Gutter Crutches**
Like other walking aids. Crutches also improves balance by increasing base of support. They are also sometimes

used for mobility in patients having arthritis to reduce weight on joints. However, crutches are not as commonly used for people for improving balance.

Chapter 8: Conclusion

The very fact that you have made it to the end of this book shows that you are a consistent person and will put in your heart and soul to improve your condition. This just shows your liveliness which is a great quality associated with people who improves their condition.

Now that you know what to do to improve your balance, you are much better positioned to improve your life condition.

Always remember that great buildings are not built in a day. It takes time. Therefore, it will also take time for your body to respond to these interventions and get stronger. Rest assured that the quality of suggestions and interventions in this book are latest, research based and presented in the simplest form to practice as soon as possible. You need to be patient and consistent. Your daily efforts will make a great difference.

Last but not the least, stay positive and have faith in yourself!

Chapter 9: Safety Checklist

1. Do not leave clutter or any other objects on the floor.
2. Make sure the area is well lit especially when you move around.
3. Keep torch nearby to use during power outages.
4. Install handrails on both sides of the stairway and be sure to use them.
5. Do not use rugs, or at least fix it to avoid slippage.
6. Install grab bars on the bathroom walls near the toilet and along the bathtub or shower.
7. Sleep on a bed that is easy for you to get in and out.
8. Do not use very low furniture which are difficult to get up from.
9. Do not keep anything far away and avoid standing on any unstable surface to reach any object.
10. Make sure any types of cords are out of the walkways.